CARNIVORE MEAL PLAN

How To Start, What To Eat, How To Succeed

Lose Weight Fast, Say Goodbye To Cravings And
Inflammation With The Definitive Carnivore Diet For
Beginners Handbook

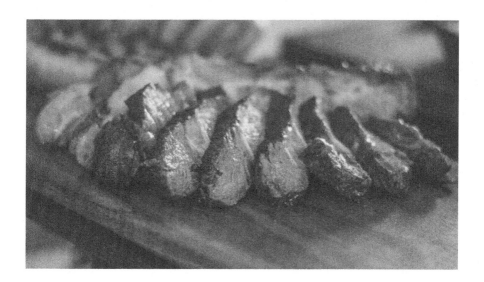

Table of Contents

Foreword

Nearly everybody needs to lose weight and remain fit, but not every person is prepared to do what will empower them to lose weight. In some different circumstances, the will is there, yet the information is missing. It is a mainstream saying that information is power, however information which is unapplied yields no outcome. Along these lines, it is more secure to state that information when applied is power.

On your weight loss journey, it is imperative to know the necessities which will yield ideal outcomes. Staying healthy, losing weight, and staying fit will consistently require some kind of stubbornness, as days will come when you will feel the need to simply eat anything. You should understand before you begin that there will be days like these and that your ability to resist the urge and defer the pleasure will determine how far your journey will last.

The carnivore diet consists only of foods of animal origin. As long as your meal participants have walked, crawled, flown, swam, or had parents, they are a "fair play" (no pun intended). You do not need to follow any rules regarding schedules, macronutrient interruptions, or portions. Simply eat when you are hungry and until you are full.

The carnivore diet itself can be at times very challenging,

especially at the beginning, but as time goes on, it will become much easier to follow. What I struggled with was building muscle and dealing with food intolerance. But I have always loved red meat and was intrigued by this diet. Since then, I have been able to complete the process myself. But I underestimated that I was involved in planning and sticking to a diet that included just meat. This guide has been compiled to avoid some of the problems that arise with eating exclusively meat. In this book, I will be guiding you through the carnivore diet, exposing its pros and cons, and providing you with useful, practical insight. Join me on this exciting journey of health and fitness!

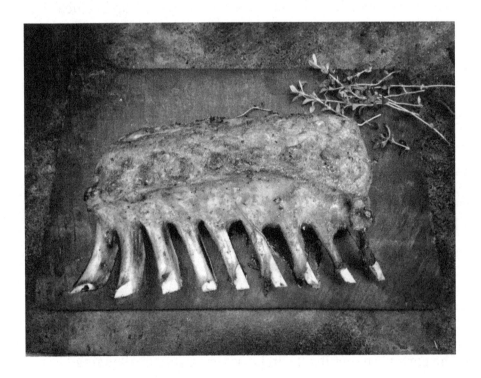

Introduction to the Carnivore Diet

THE BASICS OF THE CARNIVORE DIET

The carnivore diet consists of eating only animal foods and the total elimination of plant foods. No fruits, no vegetables, and, of course, no grains, nuts, or seeds are allowed in a strict carnivore diet. Due to the total absence of plant derived foods and, therefore, carbohydrates, the carnivore diet has also been referred to as the "Zero Carbohydrate Diet". A seemingly more striking and less aggressive name with which this diet has been recognized is imposed by a couple of Hungarian scientists who have worked with it to solve multiple diseases — cancer, irritable bowel syndrome, diabetes, etc. — and performed several studies based on it. They call this diet the "Paleolithic Carnivore Diet".

The carnivore diet is not the only nutritional regimen based on the exclusion of carbohydrates from meals. For example, the ketogenic diet is based on the same principles. However, in the keto diet, the use of carbohydrates, though still very limited, is not totally prohibited as in a strictly carnivores diet.

The carnivore diet, from the point of view of food quality, may be, as incredible as it may seem, and contrary to the common information, a superior diet. However, from a realistic perspective, particularly as regards our social life and optional nutritional freedom, I find it quite restrictive, so I won't recommend that you follow it to the letter, unless you suffer from a condition that requires it.

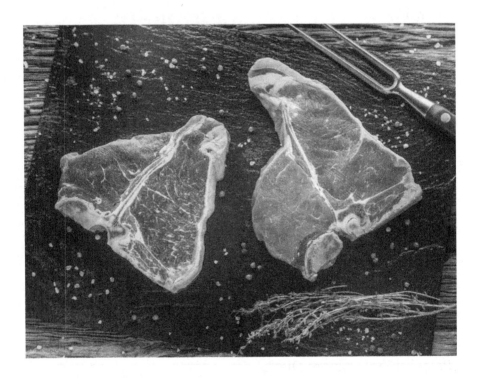

However, if you have had digestive, metabolic, and/or energy problems by including large amounts of plant-based foods — especially those with a high content of easily assimilated carbohydrates, I recommend you try this diet for at least 30 days and from there, depending on the feedback you get, adjust it to your needs, preferences, and goals by gradually reintroducing foods of plant origin, so that you get a clear picture of what works best for you in your particular case.

Plant-based foods, in general, are not an optimal source of nutrition, particularly grains, nuts/seeds, and raw vegetables, which, in addition to containing anti-nutrients that inhibit mineral absorption, can cause digestion problems.

It is best to consume most of your fat and protein requirements through animal kingdom foods — particularly from ruminants and marine creatures — due to their fat-soluble nutrient content not found in plants — Cholesterol, Vitamin D3, Vitamin A, Vitamin K2, and DHA; its greater bioavailability, and its lack of toxins.

According to our evolution, digestion, and metabolism, and in alignment with the guidelines of the healthiest diet, fruits are the best source of nutrition — especially those low in carbohydrates such as peppers, tomatoes, and cucumber — closely followed by fully cooked tubers (potato, sweet potato, cassava, etc.). Everything else — vegetables, grains, nuts, etc. — is not ideal and can be harmful. Use these vegetable food sources to meet your carbohydrate goal primarily and get most of your fats and proteins through animal products.

Chronic digestive problems are caused by things you are eating, not by things you are stopping eating - i.e., "fiber." You only need to fast for a minimum of 24 hours to corroborate this statement as a reality.

If you have problems with flatulence, intestinal inflammation, colitis, IBS, or constipation, it is best to eliminate from your diet all the foods that could be causing any of those conditions, to subsequently reintroduce them gradually — ex. one per week — and discover the culprit(s) of your discomfort. Because of its superior nutritional content and lack of elements that could disrupt good digestion, the carnivore diet is the best choice in terms of elimination diets — especially if dairy products that can be problematic in some people are also omitted.

My recommendation, based on direct experience, is regardless of your current preferences and overall current situation, you should try the carnivore diet for at least 30 days and, from there, make your decision. Maybe initially it may not seem the best option in your case. I really believe that as a method of weight loss or maintenance, it may be the perfect diet; however, to gain weight and/or display a maximum level of high physical performance — for example if you are a professional athlete — I certainly do not consider it the best choice.

Remember that any diet can help you lose or gain weight, the difference between these lies in how much this loss or gain is attributed to muscle or fat, and how sustainable this is. What will determine which diet may be ideal for you? Multiple factors: mainly your level of activity and your preferences regarding social interaction and lifestyle in general.

If you only train for health and/or aesthetics, what is the use of performing at 110% in the gym at the cost of your health and longevity? On the other hand, if you are a professional athlete, as your profession is your primary vital objective, your priorities can be the exact opposite — at least for certain periods in which your performance you want to maximize, so the inclusion of carbohydrates is something in which you shouldn't skimp.

On the other hand, if you lead a highly active social life, a diet that leaves you without eating in the multiple social events that you frequently attend may not be sustainable in the long term. Including a greater variety of foods — i.e. plants — will allow you to maintain your social life while you reach your goals of body recomposition. Finally, this is why, if one seeks to achieve an optimal balance between good physical appearance, longevity, well-being, sustainability, and health in general, carbohydrates are included — particularly around training.

Obviously, nutritional flexibility is not the same for all people and will depend mostly on your evolutionary ancestry — your inherited genetic code. Some people better assimilate carbohydrates and plant-based foods in general — for example the descendants of Chinese / Japanese — and others work best through increased proportional intake of animal foods and their fats — such as the descendants of northern Europeans.

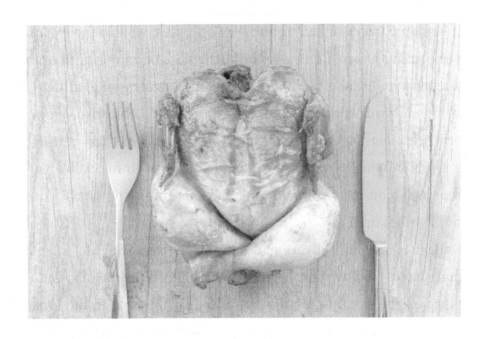

THE PROS OF THE CARNIVORE DIET

With the carnivore diet you will get the benefits of having your body in a state of ketosis. Ketosis is a metabolic process that uses stored fats as fuel. Ketosis has been associated with many benefits, including reducing the symptoms of mental health problems such as ADHD, weight loss, and muscle gain.

WEIGHT LOSS

Sugar is the standard and preferred method for light metabolic absorption, but it is also the reason for gaining weight. Then, after removing all sugar from the diet, as blood sugar levels drop, the body relies on glycogen stores. One gram of glycogen is bound with three grams of water, so you can easily lose weight by draining 4-6 kg of water.

As you well know, protein has a quite high satiating power. It's possible that after you had steak, you were quite satisfied, right? This nutrient sends a signal to your brain to warn that it has consumed the necessary amount of food and therefore reduces the craving for food. This is why people on the carnivore diet usually stop feeling so hungry and end up eating less frequently.

When you eat the same food every day, your brain loses the value of "reward". If you usually find it very rewarding to eat a great steak, after starting the carnivore diet it will feel just... usual. This can lead to an involuntary caloric restriction and lead to certain results in the body, such as:

- Decrease in the concentration of insulin and growth hormone
- Autophagy
- Reduced inflammation
- Weight loss

Reduced Inflammation

The biggest health benefit is not relying on carbohydrates, especially sugar, for energy needs. Another benefit of sugar deficiency is that it has been reported to reduce inflammation associated with arthritis. I have no personal experience with this, but I have heard of these relationships from many people I have met.

Another reason the carnivore diet reduces inflammation is it is low in waste. When we talk about "waste", we mean a substance that the body does not absorb and needs to improve intestinal transit. Therefore, in a low-residue diet, fiber-rich foods (cereals, grains, nuts, vegetables, and fruits) will have no place. A diet low in this substance is recommended in people with inflammatory bowel diseases or irritable bowel. In this case, the meat is mainly composed of proteins and fats, which leave a little residue that irritates or inflames the intestine. Of course, if you suffer from gut inflammation spicy sausages are still not a good food choice.

Muscle gain

Just following the Carnivore Diet often results in muscle building without any tinkering needed. People seamlessly achieve a body composition that makes them happy (generally beyond what they even thought possible).

For more information check the chapter "Long Lasting Benefits Of The Carnivore Diet" further along in this book.

WHAT YOU CAN EAT

All kind of meats are allowed in a carnivore diet, including:

- Beef
- Pork
- Lamb
- Poultry
- Turkey
- Duck
- Seafood
- Fish
- Various animal meats

It is desirable that all pieces of meat are as fat as possible. In addition, eggs can be added to the diet. Most people following the carnivore diet reject dairy and dairy products. It is important to remember that it is strictly forbidden to eat foods that contain grains, vegetables, fruits, mushrooms, nuts, and legumes. At first it may not be easy to follow a strict carnivore diet, but it will become easier over time. By the way you will find precious guidance to succeed on the carnivore diet in later chapters.

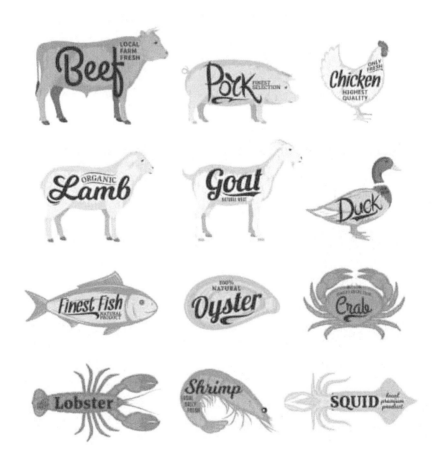

HOW MUCH AND WHEN TO EAT

Most people on a carnivore diet report it works better for them when they eat two times a day, but basically you can eat whenever you feel hungry. Also, there is no set amount of food to keep in mind for your meals. Just eat until you feel full. Having said that, a typical meal plan for a day on the carnivore diet could look something like this:

- **Breakfast**: Five slices of bacon (about 4 ounces) and one or two 100% pork sausages (3 ounces)
- **Lunch**: Grilled beef burger patty (10 ounces) with a slice of cheese
- **Dinner**: Four fresh racks of lamb (12 ounces)

The above is taken from the detailed 28-day meal plan I provide towards the end of the book. There you will find all of the information to make it to the end of your 28 day test of the carnivore diet and reap its many benefits.

For those who like to eat small snacks during the day, it is recommended to eat sausages, small pieces of meat and small fish. However, carnivores are advised to avoid unnecessary snacking when aiming for weight loss. Also, don't forget to drink enough water. You should drink frequently to reduce the possibility of digestive problems arising.

HOW TO FOLLOW THE CARNIVORE DIET

Following the carnivore diet is easy. You just have to devote yourself to eating exclusively food from the animal kingdom, with a few exceptions. First of all, since the basic principle responsible for the benefits obtained from this diet derives mainly from its carbohydrate-free nature, the consumption of animal foods with a considerable content of these such as milk, yogurt and honey is not recommended, at least not regularly, this in particular during the first 4-8 weeks of keto-adaptation - the body's adaptation to primary burning of fats and ketones instead of glucose as energy.

It should be noted that, although all types of animal meat can be consumed, due to the fat composition of certain types of animals, ideally most of your food consists of meat from ruminants (bovines, sheep, goats, etc.) and blue/fatty fish (sardines, salmon, anchovies, etc.).

The minimization of fat consumption from poultry — chicken, turkey, quail, etc. — and pork is advised due to its high content of omega 6 unsaturated fats. If you choose to consume it, prefer lean cuts of this kind of animals — skinless chicken breast, low-fat turkey ground beef, and pork chop — and, at the time of preparation, replace the missing fat with one from some ruminant — butter, beef tallow, lamb tallow, etc.

However, as a general rule, any type of animal fat is better than any type of vegetable fat — coconut oil compared to lard being a possible exception, in large part thanks to its superior nutritional content, bioavailability, and percentage composition — mostly composed of saturated, monounsaturated, and DHA fats. So, if you find yourself in a dilemma, for example, in a social event between a non-optimal animal food — ex. chicken wings — and a portion of vegetable food — ex. peanuts — you'll be a thousand times better served by opting for non-ideal animal food.

On the other hand, as a consequence of the presence in certain people of constipation, allergies, and/or general fatigue derived from the consumption of high-protein dairy products, the reduction or complete elimination of these foods — primarily cheeses and whey supplements — is suggested, at least in the initial stages of introduction to this type of diet. However, the inclusion of dairy derivatives with almost zero amounts of protein, such as butter, cream, and cream cheese, is advised if a substantial intake of fats by pure ingestion of meat products cannot be achieved.

After the initial period of adaptation (1-3 months), the consumption of milk proteins can be added progressively, of course, if none of the symptoms described previously — constipation, inflammation, tiredness, etc. — occurs at the beginning of reintroduction. In the end we can define the optimal foods to be included in this diet:

- All kinds of meats — especially ruminants (cow, sheep, goat, etc.).

- All kinds of fish and shellfish — especially fatty ones (salmon, sardines, anchovies, etc.).
- Low carb dairy products if they are well tolerated — cheeses, cream, butter, etc.

Additionally, the consumption of organs - liver, brains, kidneys, etc. — bone broth, and "gelatinous" connective tissue periodically is highly recommended. This is mostly to prevent any potential nutritional deficiency — folate, vitamin C, DHA, etc.; get extra electrolytes — calcium, magnesium, potassium, etc. — and maintain a good glycine:methionine intake ratio.

If you want a simple diet that meets all the characteristics of a properly implemented carnivore diet, the "Steak and Eggs" diet will work for you as it consists of only three foods in this category: steak, eggs - which replace consumption of organ meat to some degree, and butter. Of course, you will have to skip the "cheat day" suggested by its creator, since originally this can include foods that your butcher can not be a supplier of. The advantage and greater difference of this diet compared to its more conservative version are that in this, you do not have to worry about consuming "too much protein" — and much fewer carbohydrates since it is certain that you will not be consuming any.

POSSIBLE CONS AND RISKS

The carnivore diet involves eating almost exclusively meat on a daily basis. This means that it is high in protein, high in fat, and low in carbohydrates. This is inconsistent with traditional nutritional wisdom that contributed to the spread of vegetarianism, such as "you need to eat lots of vegetables, dietary fiber, and whole grains." Carnivores are expected to have problems such as high cholesterol, digestive problems, and weight gain. But conventional wisdom is not always accurate. My personal advice is to try for yourself for at least a month and see the benefits you can get. This book will help you achieve exactly that.

RISK OF NUTRIENT DEFICIT

Although there are no studies that negatively and categorically point out the carnivore diet as dangerous to health, it is true that it lacks the contribution of many nutrients commonly deemed essential to enjoy good functioning, and one must be fully aware of that before trying the diet.

There are four micronutrients that are difficult to achieve on a diet based on meat only:

- **Vitamin C**. In an antioxidant that stimulates the functioning of immune cells.

- **Vitamin E**. Prevents oxidation of lipids and lipoproteins.
- **Vitamin K2**. It reduces the calcification of blood vessels.
- **Calcium**. It is a necessary mineral to have healthy bones, as well as to achieve muscle contraction and nerve transmission.

LACK OF BENEFICIAL PHYTONUTRIENTS

Phytonutrients are chemicals that plants produce to protect themselves from environmental threats, such as insects or diseases. Interestingly, these phytonutrients have health benefits. And many will know them with the name of curcumin, beta-carotene, quercetin or resveratrol. Those who defend the carnivore diet comment that phytonutrients are toxic to humans, and that the ideal is to eliminate them completely from our diet. For other people, many of these "toxins" make us much more resistant immunologically.

RISK OF LIVER OVERLOAD

When our body does not eat enough hydrates and fats, the liver can produce glucose from proteins (gluconeogenesis).

This causes nitrogen wastes to be created that have to be eliminated through the kidneys. The process is completely normal, and our body is designed for it, the problem appears when you have to handle very large quantities. Exceeding more than 40% daily protein intake would be above the safe limit.

RISK OF HORMONAL IMBALANCE

There is still no research that reports on the long-term effect of a carnivore diet on hormones, thyroid function, and fertility. In the case of pregnant women, it is shown that a low carbohydrate diet can negatively influence fertility. Carbohydrates are an important nutrient in thyroid function since insulin stimulates thyroid hormones.

LOW VITAMIN C INTAKE

Organ meats and eggs are about your only option apart from supplementation to get the Vitamin C you need. Vitamin C is vital for repairing our body's tissues and helps reduce the chance of chronic diseases.

Loss of Good Bacteria

Many carnivore evangelists note that intestinal issues are resolved after beginning a carnivore diet. This may be true due to the elimination of typical inflammatory foods like sugar, lactose, or anything else your body may be sensitive too. The issue is if good bacteria is eliminated overtime as well, which could cause a variety of digestion issues.

Excessive Sodium and Saturated Fats

Eating only meat and dairy will almost certainly increase your intake of sodium and saturated fats. Excess sodium can contribute to headaches, swelling, and kidney disease, and excess saturated fats can increase your risk of a stroke.

The Origins Of The Carnivore Diet

It may seem a bit "anecdotal" and lacking in scientific basis, but most of the mainly carnivorous cultures, especially those directly descended from the Paleolithic period, are characterized by their superior height, musculature and brain volume, this, in contrast to the cultures who based their diet mainly on food provided by agriculture, for example the Maya. What is the reason behind this difference?

Most likely the nutritional superiority of the diet in general: high-quality proteins, animal fats and micronutrients with much better bioavailability; better digestibility - low in "fiber" and anti-nutrients, and less ingestion of toxins - phytochemicals and pesticides.

For example, the Mongolian culture led by Genghis Khan swept through Asian cultures, which surpassed the Mongols in a proportion of at least 2 to 1, most likely due to their physical superiority acquired through their diet, which was mostly based on Meat and dairy products.

The Mongols of that time were much more muscular, tall, and stronger than their undernourished Asian opponents, short in stature, and deformed dentures attributed to a diet high in carbohydrates — especially grains — and low in animal foods — high protein quality, cholesterol-based fats, and vitamins B12, K2, D3, and A. Certainly, the merit of Genghis Khan as leader and military strategist cannot be ignored in his ability to conquer, but it would be a mistake not to consider the element of bodily supremacy of the members of his army. Similarly, cultures such as the Masai, the Inuit, and the Chukotka are recognized for their enviable physical strength, formidable muscles and height, and their attractive body and dental symmetry. Like the Mongols of ancient times, these societies maintain a diet based mainly on animal products: meat, fish, dairy products, eggs, blood, etc.

On the contrary, so far, it is not known of a healthy society that is or has been totally vegetarian. Individuals recognized for their contribution in the field of nutritional demographic study and their relationship with social body welfare such as Catherine Shanahan, Loren Cordain, and Weston Price have noted similar results: the higher the consumption of quality animal food in a culture, especially those derived from ruminants and fish, the better the development of infants and the general health of society in particular. Are we evolutionarily designed to consume mostly animal products and their derivatives?

THE EVOLUTIONARY LOGIC AND THE CARNIVORE DIET

The Paleolithic Period is the oldest period in which man, as he is known today — "Homo Sapiens," has been alive, and the longest of the Stone Age. It dates from 2,000,000 BC to 10,000 BC. The people of the Paleolithic Period lived simple lives, which consisted mainly of survival and reproduction. Man's life was simply to hunt, eat and survive, while the woman's job was food collection and childcare. With the birth of agriculture the Paleolithic period ended, giving entrance to the Neolithic. The food sources of human hunter-gatherers of this period included animals and plants that were part of the natural environment in which these humans lived, often meat from animal organs, such as the liver, kidneys, and brain was consumed. These humans consumed few dairy foods or carbohydrate-rich plant foods such as legumes, tubers, or cereals, especially during the ice age, in which plant-based foods were scarce — if not nonexistent, and the emphasis on consumption of animal products had to be emphasized.

Current research indicates that, during the Paleolithic, two-thirds of the energy was derived from the food of animal origin. The fat content of the diet was similar to that of today, but the proportion of the types of fat consumed was different: the ratio of Omega-6 to Omega-3 was about 3:1 in drastic comparison with the average proportion of 12:1 of today's diet. The few carbohydrates that were consumed came purely from fruits — especially berries (strawberries, blueberries, raspberries, etc.), milk, and vegetables. In addition to this, there is the theory that we humans are the only mammals that cool primarily through our ability to sweat, a mechanism developed to run for long distances and hunt. Sweat, by cooling the body, allows us to run long distances so that we can chase our hunting prey.

On the other hand, why is the dog's best friend a fully carnivore animal? If you have one of these fantastic animals as a companion, you will have noticed that no matter how much you try to educate it differently, whenever you sit down to eat it comes close so that you share it with your food — particularly if what you will eat is of animal origin.

In fact, most dogs, regardless of their breed or origin, intuitively — you don't need to show it to them, they give you the leg or put their face on your knee to ask for some food.

Dogs are the domesticated version of wolves. Through their evolution, they have graduated from active hunters to mostly passive hunters. Due to the reduction in their fierce appearance compared to that of the common wolf, it has been easier for the human being to adopt them as part of the family. Thanks to this, dogs no longer have to worry about acquiring their food through active hunting, but they help the human in this arduous task or, as is the most current case, they do not even help him get it, they only receive it. A carnivore pet for a carnivore animal: is that the reason why we get along so well?

PLANTS ARE A BAD SOURCE OF NUTRIENTS

The reality is that, contrary to popular belief, plants, but especially vegetables, are a bad source of nutrients, at least in their natural form — raw. Although no one denies that theoretically there are vegetables that have an outstanding micro-nutritional content — spinach, broccoli, kale, etc. — the reality is that these, in addition to being accompanied by other harmful compounds for their consumer, have elements that inhibit their absorption, so, for more vitamins and minerals they contain, if they are not fully absorbed they cannot be considered relevant. In addition, all plants — without exception — lack essential nutrients that can only be acquired through animal products, such as Vitamin D3, Vitamin K2, Vitamin A, Cholesterol, DHA, Vitamin B12, and a complete protein profile — they do not contain all the essential amino acids. It is thanks to this that followers of vegetarian diets often present marked deficiencies of these key components.

ANTI-NUTRIENTS AND PESTICIDES

The plant's natural anti-nutrients and pesticides block the absorption of nutrients contained in the plant and can cause us other problems. Many of the famous "Phyto-nutrients" — which actually used to be categorized as Phytochemicals, are really pesticides designed to harm the insects that try to consume the plant in question. They are not nutrition, and they are protected. That a phytochemical demonstrates killing isolated cancer cells "in vitro" does not show anything about its potential to empower our health. It only shows that it can kill cells, healthy or mutated.

FATTY ACID COMPOSITION

Most plant-based foods are high in omega 6 polyunsaturated

fats, and those that contain a higher proportion of omega 3 contain it in a form not easily assimilated by the body and, generally, in the company of other compounds harmful to your body. Given that high consumption of omega 6, especially that of plant origin, is something highly detrimental to your well-being, we can realize that eating primarily food from the plant kingdom is not ideal.

In addition, no plant-based foods, even those that contain a higher proportion of pro-testosterone fats — saturated and monounsaturated — such as coconut, cocoa, and avocado, contain cholesterol. Contrary to what the popular narrative dictates, having low levels of total cholesterol is not something positive, but harmful. Cholesterol is essential for the proper functioning of the human body — particularly the nervous, immune, and hormonal system, to the point that, if not consumed, the body looks for ways to produce it on its own — that is, independently. How much of this element you consume, your body will keep a similar volume in blood.

Cholesterol intake is not something you should avoid, but quite the contrary, its consumption in a person who can process you in a healthy way is something I feel safe in encouraging. Of course, if your hormonal profile, immune system, and overall health, you want to maximize. Basically, the carnivore diet is an improved ketogenic diet: no anti-nutrients — fiber, pesticides, digestive function inhibitors; with higher content of fat-soluble essential nutrients —

Cholesterol, Vitamin D3, Vitamin A, Vitamin K2, and DHA; and with an optimal proportional fat balance — a breakdown composed mostly of saturated and monounsaturated fats (pro-vitality, pro-testosterone, and pro-longevity fats).

THE VITAMIN C AND ANTIOXIDANTS DILEMMA

The only vitamin of which animal products are not a good source is the famous vitamin C, whose deficiency is the direct cause of the condition called scurvy. What about antioxidants? If plants are the best source of vitamin C and the only source of antioxidants, how come there are still thousands of people like Shawn Baker, Dany Vega, and Amber O'Hearn who have been years, not only surviving, but thriving without consuming any plant food? This without counting the current cultures that follow a similar diet — Masai, Inuit, Chukotka, etc.; and the long glacial period in which humans had to feed themselves purely from hunting — plant foods, due to freezing, did not exist.

- Is ascorbic acid — the scientific name of "Vitamin C" — really an essential nutrient for every animal?
- Are there particular conditions that affect the need for Vitamin C and, therefore, its essentiality?

- Can we maintain good health — free of scurvy — if we avoid certain compounds that increase the intake requirement of this element and consume foods that contain it somewhat correctly?

As for the aforementioned antioxidant power of this famous vitamin, do we need to consume antioxidants in general, or is our body able to produce them endogenously, by itself? Are exogenously acquired antioxidants — which are consumed — really used in the first place?

Let's see what scientific research thinks about these questions:

- **Evidence #1**: Vitamin C is not an essential nutrient for every animal, but for humans, it is, since, like other primates, and unlike other mammals, we cannot synthesize it in the liver.
- **Evidence #2**: Carbohydrate intake increases the requirement of vitamin C in humans since these compounds compete with each other directly in the body. The more carbohydrates we consume, the greater our requirement in the body of this compound, so that, in a diet of almost zero content of these, the necessary vitamin C can be easily acquired through foods with minimum content.

- **Evidence #3**: In an old expedition, in which scurvy entered into action, it was found that the consumption of fresh meat, due to its vitamin C content, was able to cure this discomfort. In addition, when experimenting, it has been found that 10mg daily — easily obtained by fresh meat (especially the liver) — is sufficient to prevent a deficiency, while more than 70mg does not provide an additional benefit.

- **Evidence #4**: Glutathione, which is more actively synthesized during ketosis by humans, in addition to promoting the reuse of existing vitamin C, is an antioxidant with similar actions — if not more potent — than vitamin C. On the other hand, uric acid, another endogenous antioxidant, has similar functions.

- **Evidence #5**: Non-nutritive ingested antioxidants, those that are not a vitamin or mineral, are not as well used by our body as has been so commonly reported. Most of them are not absorbed, transformed, or simply excreted.

In addition to this, high carbohydrate intake increases the body's overall oxidation, so the reduction in its intake — by following a carnivore diet, for example — reduces the need for antioxidants that counteract excessive oxidation, so your intake loses relevance.

A carnivore diet primarily based on fresh and carbohydrate-free ruminant meat has sufficient vitamin C content, and keeps the body's overall oxidation under control without acquiring antioxidants through ingestion. The necessary antioxidant work is exercised by the body naturally endogenously, therefore, it is fully compatible with excellent health.

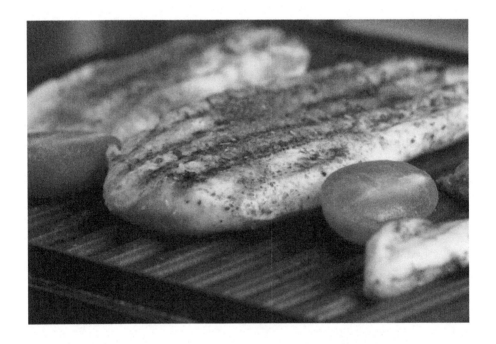

Understanding The Digestive Function

Humans, for many years, have been primarily carnivores, to the point that many researchers have proposed that, due to cooperative hunting, our brain developed so much compared to other primates. Biologically, our teeth evolutionarily designed to tear meat, our highly acidic non-fermentable digestive tract, and our gallbladder designed to dissolve a high amount of dietary fat prove it.

Is it normal for an animal to suffer from dental cavities, stomach indigestion, malodorous flatulence, abdominal pain, and irregular bowel movements — constipation and/or diarrhea — often? Of course not. These problems are derived from poor digestion, certainly caused by the ingestion of food that does not allow the digestive system of the animal in question to perform its proper function.

THE HUMAN DIGESTIVE SYSTEM

We do not need to eat plant-based foods, and we probably work better without them. Our digestive system is primarily designed to process animal meat. First of all our teeth, due to their structure optimized for tearing the meat and their totally vertical movement during chewing — and not circular like that of a herbivore — are ideal for the consumption of food of animal origin. Just compare your teeth with those of your dog and then with those of a cow, horse, or sheep. Which ones are more similar? Our stomach, like other carnivores such as canines, is highly acidic, which makes it ideal for the digestion of foods high in protein — not "fiber." Our small intestine, unlike herbivores that ferment plants in a second stage - ruminants ferment cellulose ingested first in their rumen — is much longer than our large intestine. In fact, we can live without the large intestine without any problems, since it does not provide us with additional benefits in the absorption of nutrients — herbivores, on the other hand, cannot live without their large intestine because in that case they would be malnourished. The bacteria found in our large intestine, being mainly non-fermentative, usually balance and function better when fed with residual fats and proteins, non-fermentable and non-assimilable carbohydrates — i.e., "fiber."

You don't need to take my word for it, take a test. Even just following the carnivore diet for a week, do your digestive problems persist? We are certainly not herbivores, probably omnivores, but definitely carnivores.

THE OPTIMAL METABOLISM

Since I remember, every time I eat a substantial amount of carbohydrates (> 50gr), I usually suffer from symptoms related to hypoglycemia — sweating, trembling, tiredness, etc; especially if they come from low-fiber starches — flour, white rice, tortillas, etc. In fact, the only proven benefit of fiber is that when consumed in conjunction with carbohydrates — as they naturally come, it helps reduce the glycemic index of food so that the carbohydrates consumed are more slowly absorbed — ex. The glycemic and insulinogenic peak will not be the same when consuming a banana compared to a piece of wheat flour bread. Certainly, humans, or rather, all mammals, are not designed to consume large amounts of glucose — especially in isolation.

Even herbivores do not consume a large amount of carbohydrates on a regular basis as is mistakenly believed — in nature, the food primarily consumed by other primates is not bananas (or really any other fruit high in sugar); but, by fermenting the fiber contained in plants, they acquire substantial amounts of fatty acids — particularly saturated short chain.

In fact, captive gorillas fed primarily with fruits instead of usable low-carb vegetables often suffer from diseases associated with humanity today - cardiovascular diseases, cancer, diabetes, etc.; something that does not happen and stops happening when they are free or are given adequate food — based on vegetables high in fiber and low in glucose/fructose. In the case of humans, a healthy body usually maintains about 8gr of sugar/blood glucose — the equivalent of 2 teaspoons of sugar. A level higher than this is identified as toxic to the body. High blood glucose peaks usually cause damage to cells, especially those belonging to the nervous system.

Indeed, most of the discomforts experienced by diabetics — gangrene, glaucoma, dry skin, etc. — come from high blood glucose levels chronically. Imagine what happens when you ingest a large amount of easily-assimilated highly-processed carbohydrates — flour, pure sugar, white rice, etc. What do you think your body does?

That's right, when that large amount of glucose is digested and thrown into the blood, the body enters a state of emergency and, as a contingency, secretes an equivalent amount of insulin to lower the very high and harmful level of blood glucose caused by your indulgence, which generally causes a disproportionate reaction of this hormone and leaves the body with a lower level than the ideal as a consequence, that is, in a state of slight hypoglycemia — especially if you are someone relatively resistant to the action of insulin. This phenomenon caused by the consumption of a large number of carbohydrates — especially in the form of starches, is commonly known as "rebound" or "reactive" hypoglycemia.

Bounce hypoglycemia is the cause of excessive tiredness, brain fog, and drowsiness, similar to that experienced after ingestion of a large amount of food — something that does not happen if the food is based on fats and protein instead of carbohydrates.

In addition to this, because your blood glucose level becomes too low, your carbohydrate appetite is immediately and acutely presented in order to return the blood sugar level to stable levels. This is why you usually suffer from hunger — sometimes even on a full stomach — after having had for breakfast your "cereal with light milk" 2-3 hours before. On the other hand, if you have a high-fat and low-carb breakfast even with the same caloric content, this does not happen — after a "steak and eggs" breakfast at 7 am you can refrain from eating food until 2-3 pm without any problem. Contrary to what doctors, personal trainers, and nutritionists/dietitians tell you, this is NOT normal. Excessive tiredness and appetite after feeding should not happen. The advice of having a meal every 2-3 hours to maintain blood glucose levels should not exist.

Finally, in addition to the fact that multiple cycles of reactive hypoglycemia — hyperglycemia followed by hypoglycemia — damage the cells, the nervous system, and the immune system, it is very likely that these too, if they occur chronically, cause increased resistance to insulin — prediabetes. Ketosis may or may not be the ideal metabolic state of humanity. What is absolutely clear is that following this diet, or any other low carb diet, such as carnivore, avoiding high blood glucose fluctuations will prevent fatigue/heaviness after feeding, the possible damage to your cells caused by the hyperglycemia, premature aging derived high oxidation, high glycation — the combination of protein and glucose "harden" the binding between cells. To lose weight, speaking of most sedentary people or who exercise for health, appearance, and/or entertainment — i.e., people who are not athletes — a low carb diet seems to be the best way to go, particularly if you have relatively high insulin resistance, as reported in multiple studies on the subject, in millions of success stories around the world, as well as in my personal experience.

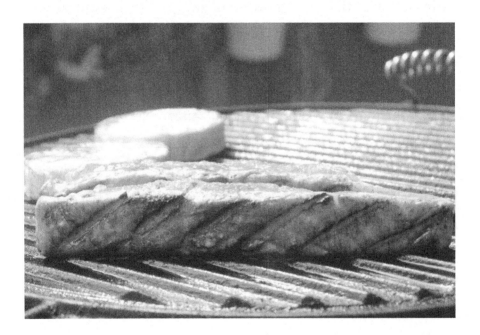

Meat Types And Allowed Foods

Meat fans may find the carnivore diet very tempting. Although there is no official definition, the carnivore diet is the one that includes foods that walk, swim, or fly. Plant-based foods, such as vegetables, nuts, and seeds, are not allowed.

ALLOWED FOODS

- Red meat (beef, pork or lamb), with special emphasis on the fattier cuts
- Poultry
- Fish
- Lard
- Tallow
- Salt and pepper

Allowed Beverages

- Bone broth
- Water (with or without carbonation or minerals)

SIDES AND EXCEPTIONS

These will depend on how strict the diet is:

- Eggs
- Milk
- Yogurt
- Cheese
- Coffee
- Tea

PROHIBITED FOODS

Everything that is not meat:

- Vegetables
- Fruit
- Seeds
- Nuts
- Legumes
- Bread
- Pasta
- Grains

KNOW YOUR FOODS

BEEF

Steak, hamburgers, and red meat, in general, are the main food sources for carnivores. Since you are not eating carbohydrates or any type of vegetable food, it is essential that you consume enough calories to keep your energy high, so fatter cuts of meat are best. Poultry and organ meats are also good, as are processed meat products like bacon and sausage as long as they are handcrafted. The best cuts of beef to eat are:

- Steaks
- Roasts
- Ground beef

If you're doing the carnivore diet on a budget (I'm giving you 6 money saving tips on the carnivore diet in a later chapter), go for the ground beef and roasts over steak. However, experiment with fat intake because with ground beef you may be getting substantially less fat. Compared to other animals, ruminants and beef have a better omega 6 : omega 3 ratio which affects inflammation. Pork bacon has 8000mg of Linoleic acid whereas there is only 159mg for beef. Beef is also much higher in almost every single nutrient than pork bacon.

	100g Beef Steak	100g Pork Bacon
	RDA %	RDA %
Vitamin A (Retinol)	1.50%	0%
Vitamin B1	8%	7%
Vitamin B2	13%	4%
Vitamin B3	52%	7%
Vitamin B5	5%	0%
Vitamin B6	12%	0%
Vitamin B7	3%	0%
Vitamin B9	1%	0%
Vitamin B12	164%	7%
Vitamin C	Depends	0%
Vitamin D	0%?	0%
Vitamin E	4%	6%
Vitamin K2	19%	0%
Sodium	4%	0%
Potassium	9%	0%
Calcium	1%	0%
Magnesium	6%	0%
Phosphorous	22%	1%
Sulfur	183mg	7mg
Chloride	5%	0%
Iron	16%	1%
Zinc	47%	1%
Copper	6%	1%
Iodine	0%	0%
EPA O3	12mg	169mg
DHA O3	0mg	0mg
Oleic O9	2504mg	37786mg
Linoleic O6	159mg	8030mg
Linolenic O3	66mg	761mg

Fish

Any type is good, but again, fatter types like salmon and sardines are the smartest choices.

Bone Broth

Fully allowed and recommended. Fatty meat products Lard and other high-fat foods derived from meat are allowed and always used to replace vegetable oils whenever necessary.

Whole Eggs

You can eat eggs, since they are animal products. Most importantly, eggs don't have any carbohydrates. Carbohydrates are the nutrients that destroy you as a human. If you're not fat adapted yet and still in ketosis, you'll remain in ketosis if you eat eggs which is another goal. Cholesterol and fat are in the yolk, that is the color of gold for a reason: it's gold for our bodies. One of the largest diet myths in society today is the intake of Cholesterol. We've been taught by society and so-called "expert doctors" that Cholesterol is bad.
Another health-damaging diet myth is on saturated fat: we've been told that saturated fat is bad and unsaturated fat is good. This again simply isn't true. Eating saturated fat is what your body needs for fuel. Your body either uses carbohydrates or fat

for fuel. Your body wants to use fat for fuel, but if you're eating carbs, then you won't. You will use carbs for fuel and the fat will stack up and will show you the excess fat that is being built up when you look in the mirror.

Since intolerances to these are actually quite common, I personally recommend going without for at least some time. After removing them for a time, if you desire, you can reintroduce them later and evaluate how you feel. When buying eggs, prefer those from farm raised, natural, organic, non-hormonal fed chickens. Find a farmer that will sell you eggs, meat and raw milk. That's the best way to get your food.

SPICES

Salt and pepper are your best friends, as are parsley, garlic, mustard, and various herbs and spices that technically do not qualify as of animal origin. Most sugar-free condiments do not contain substances that cause digestive problems in most people, so I see no harm in using them just because they come from plants (especially since people normally appreciate condiments in small portions). Still, due to its fat content, meat - particularly red meat - is quite tasty in its own right, so you will probably find that salt, pepper, or small amounts of butter provide the flavor you want without the need to add something else.

COFFEE

Coffee is a plant extract and caffeine is a natural insecticide. But, if you are a coffee drinker, I recommend you keep drinking it for the first 30 days, since getting through the carnivore adaptation plus caffeine withdrawal would be too much.

Coffee is an allowed exception for most carnivores, although I recommend starting tapering towards the end of the month after adaptation symptoms have resolved somewhat. Though most people do fine with coffee, for some people cutting it makes all the difference. It's worth it to find out if that's you.

DAIRY PRODUCTS

Cheese, yogurt, and butter all come from animals and are technically permissible, although most carnivores seem to omit or at least limit them. This is usually due to people who discover the carnivore diet as a consequence of the keto diet, in which milk and yogurt are generally not allowed due to their lactose (sugar) content. Since one of the goals of a carnivore diet is to eliminate nutrients that your body may not be able to process optimally, you should try dairy foods one at a time and in small doses to see how you handle them. You can feel better without dairy products.

SUPPLEMENTS

None. Although products like whey protein and creatine come from animals, there is virtually no need to supplement them in this case. Eating exclusively animal foods ensures that you meet your daily protein needs, and relying on red meat, which is rich in creatine naturally, leaves little reason for additional supplementation. Working-out carnivores report consuming coffee or caffeine supplements for an energy-boosting pre-exercise (despite the fact that it is not an animal product). If you are afraid of not getting enough micronutrients from your food, seek individualized nutritional monitoring.

Long Lasting Benefits Of The Carnivore Diet

Here are all the benefits I have personally experienced while following the carnivore diet.

IMPROVED DIGESTIVE FUNCTION

Since my childhood, I have experienced frequent episodes of indigestion, intestinal inflammation and gas, coupled with an intermittence between constipation and mild diarrhea. Fortunately, most of these symptoms decreased when introducing the carnivore diet, but each time I consumed a considerable amount of foods high in soluble fiber - broccoli, cauliflower, etc. these symptoms returned. The reason for this: our digestive system, is primarily carnivore, is not designed to process large amounts of fiber in general, but particularly fermentable.

As we have seen, since our intestinal flora is mainly non-fermentative, the assimilation of large quantities of non-digestible vegetable matter, in our case, is not something natural. What hurts your gut, what makes your stomach swell and causes you to emit foul-smelling gases, cannot be natural, and I think there isn't much to disprove in that statement.

In addition to the fact that my body no longer produces so many intestinal gases in general — so inflammation and pain are no longer a problem; the few that are produced have no smell — literally. And that's how it should be.

Following this diet, I experienced the best digestive function of my life.

BETTER SLEEP QUALITY

Thanks to this diet, I sleep more deeply and, consequently, I sleep less time and get up cooler. Previously, I used to sleep 7-9 hours and get up tired. Following this diet, 5-7 hours of sleep - usually 6 - are more than enough, so I get up earlier, more rested and maintain this well-being for longer throughout the day. In other words, as Arnold Schwarzenegger once suggested, "I sleep faster".

Another positive aspect related is that since I follow this diet, I have not had a nightmare, or I have risen sweating profusely, something that even in the keto diet happened. I attribute this difference to the absence of usable residual carbohydrates, but to a greater extent to the total absence of anti-nutrients, gastro-inflammatory "fiber" and unsaturated fats of vegetable origin — especially omega 6. Basically, every time I go to bed with the intention of resting, I sleep like a baby.

GREATER ENERGY STABILITY

Thanks to this diet, my energy levels are much more stable throughout the day. With the keto diet I was on, my energy levels had already benefited a lot, but by switching to the carnivore diet completely, of course, my energy has never been better - also bear in mind that I was already up to a high standard. What is the reason for this improvement? The cause is most likely the absence of drastic spikes in blood glucose and subsequent hypoglycemia when the exaggerated action of insulin comes into play, along with the increase in the primary male hormone - testosterone.

BETTER TRAINING PERFORMANCE

Thanks to the increase in energy described in the previous point, my workouts, after a certain period of adaptation, have seen if not a benefit - even if I believe so - the maintenance of the ability to lift weight. An added bonus is that since when I train by burning fat and ketones instead of glucose, I'm not "hitting rock bottom" or feeling hypoglycemic in the middle of training, anymore.

Also, if you are like me and, during the adaptations associated with this diet, choose to do long walks to reflect, meditate or think, you can do it for hours without feeling any fatigue or discomfort - it's like having infinite energy.

QUICKER TRAINING RECOVERY

My post-workout recovery has never been better. My muscles no longer ache after having stimulated them intensely — not so much, not for so long. Sometimes I don't even feel trained enough since the usual pain I experienced before is nonexistent even though I continue to lift heavy. Thanks to this, I am now able to train, if I wish, almost daily.

GREATER MOOD, COGNITIVE, AND EMOTIONAL STABILITY

No more drowsiness after lunch — or any other meal. No more drastic fluctuations in my mood or cognitive ability. No more deficiencies in my emotional intelligence. Now, for most of the day — or at least the most socially active part of it — I can keep my ability to think at a high level and keep my emotionality controlled by my rationality — a highly masculine and beneficial trait — so it's easier to lead an increasingly positive, well focused and stoic life.

APPETITE SUPPRESSION

It is very clear to me that, at least in my experience, the carnivore diet is not a good diet to gain weight — especially if the weight gain is difficult for you, this due to its marked ability to decrease appetite. Following this diet, you can eat two times a day without starving or experiencing substantial energy losses. This is why, if your current goal is to lose weight, any low carb diet, but especially the carnivore diet, is a highly recommended option.

No More Cravings

Once you have satisfied your hunger through a good steak, eggs, or the combination of both, the craving for muffins, candies, chocolates, and really any other food, will cease to exist.

Due to the superior micronutrient content and bioavailability of meat, combined with its high level of high-quality proteins and saturated and monounsaturated fats based on cholesterol — all these elements being natural appetite suppressants — your hunger and cravings for another type of more "fun" meals will be reduced to zero.

No More Seasonal Allergies

Although the keto diet had already helped me a lot with this problem, the carnivore or "Zero Carbs" diet took it a step further. All my life, before getting involved with the carnivore diet, I had suffered from symptoms related to the common cold (profuse mucus, tearing, sneezing, etc.) in the mornings at certain times of the year, this, most likely due to an autoimmune response to the pollen or dust. This has never happened to me again, not even a single day, regardless of the season - winter / spring. Now, without morning allergies, I feel healthy every day.

IMMUNE SYSTEM IMPROVEMENTS

In addition to the benefits described above, it has been years — approximately since I began fasting intermittently daily (which induces the state of ketosis momentarily) — without having had flu/cold symptoms and, now that I remember, no other type of lasting infection. Because my body does not experience exaggerated glucose fluctuations — which lower the defenses, my immune system is stronger than ever.

ACNE REDUCTION

Being on a diet with almost no carbohydrate content, a key point in the treatment of acne, will put your acne in partial or total remission. In fact, due to the roots of this pathology, one of the fastest ways to recognize a person suffering from a high level of insulin resistance is to look at his/her skin - in fact, this condition shouldn't be something "normal" outside of puberty. It is for this reason that societies that base their diets on whole foods do not usually present this condition. This, due to the lack of a large number of usable carbohydrates in the diet, but also due to the drastic increase in the intake of nutrients that prevent this disease and which can only be obtained in sufficient quantities through foods of animal origin - Vitamin A, Vitamin D3 and DHA.

By following this diet, if you currently suffer from acne, you will see that the lesions related to this condition will be very rare or even nonexistent, especially if you also eliminate the dairy products that usually cause problems in some people.

ENDURING SATISFACTION

Although it seems initially that this will be a boring and unsatisfactory diet, believe me, it will not be, especially if you are keen on eating beef primarily. I've always said it and in this circumstance I confirm it, if there is one food that I could eat in all my meals, every day, for the rest of my life, that would undoubtedly be beef, particularly if it comes in the form of succulent, high-fat steaks. I just don't get tired of eating it, and, according to multiple reports of long time followers of this diet, mine is not an extraordinary case but the norm. There is no doubt that the human body is a highly sophisticated organism, it knows what is convenient for it and, generally, it induces you to give it what is best for it — beef. However, if you don't get full satisfaction from eating beef continuously — which I doubt, you have multiple other options to provide "variety" to this diet. Starting with the vast diversity of existing ruminants - goat, sheep, deer, lama, bison, etc. - and continuing with any other animal that interests you to taste — fish, shellfish, pork, etc.

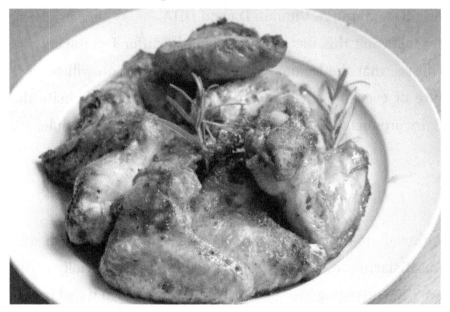

How To Complete The First Month And Continue

There can be many challenges when starting a meat-based diet. Below you can find out what these challenges are and some strategies that, based on my direct personal experience, have proven effective in overcoming them. Identifying these potential challenges ahead of time and planning your strategy to overcome them will make it easier and less stressful to face them.

TIPS TO MAKE IT THROUGH THE FIRST MONTH

- **Consult your doctor before you start**

Let's start with an important caveat. Each person's body is slightly different and reacts differently to different foods. That doesn't mean the results aren't beneficial, but it's best to take any diet with a grain of salt and consult a doctor before trying it. Take a blood test before you start your journey, so you can measure the effect of the diet 2-3 months later. Consult your doctor or nutritionist before trying.

If you decide to try, be aware of the changes in your energy, digestion, and weight. We are all different. While many people report benefiting from meat eating patterns, others may have problems.

- **Take it easy**

The first week for me was hard. Expect changes in hunger, energy, and concentration. Start with a less busy week. Work remotely. Take a rest. Sleep a little more.

- **Don't quit when you don't feel good**

You'll likely experience fatigue, headaches, and other flu-like symptoms during the first week of the diet. This is a normal part of the process as your body is getting used to using fats for energy rather than carbs. The symptoms you may experience due to your body's natural response to carbohydrate restriction and the elimination of addictive agents and chemicals include: brain fog, headache, chills, sore throat, digestive issues, dizziness, irritability, bad breath/smells, bad taste in mouth (metallic), dry mouth, cravings (sugar), muscle soreness, nausea, diarrhea, poor focus, decreased performance and energy, rapid heart rate, insomnia, night sweats, and nocturia (peeing a lot at night). Being fully aware of the adaptation process is key to avoid freaking out when not feeling good and quitting.

- **Be prepared for changes in appetite**

Some days went on for hours without hunger. One day, at 10 in the morning, I was hungry (after having breakfast), in fact, I was starving and longed for a great meal. Make sure you have access to carnivore-friendly foods throughout the day until you find the right amount to eat throughout the day.

After a few days I lost my appetite for steak. I don't know if I bought a wrong cut or cooked it poorly, but as you can imagine, it's very hard not to feel like steak when your diet is steak. The cheese helped. I ate a lot of it in the first week. Keep it if you need it. If you need to make an exception to the rule, and I did it the first week, try eating something that's not too far off the carnivore diet, like peanut butter. Peanut butter isn't part of the diet, but it's not as bad as Twinkies. It is very tasty, so it helps you overcome your desire for something that is bad for you.

- **Eat out properly**

The good news is that unless you are at a vegan restaurant, there is meat on about every menu. Just ask for a steak or a burger patty with nothing else. I've found many fast-food joints are extremely accommodating and fair priced.

POSSIBLE TRANSITORY SIDE EFFECTS

During the adaptation phase to achieve full ketosis, there can be temporary, unwanted side effects.

- **Brain Fog**

Brain fog, or lack of mental concentration is very common and annoying. Basically, the digestive system sends signals to the brain. "Hey, what are you doing? I'm hungry here." In human history, stress and anxiety were a natural reaction of the brain because getting food was very dangerous before it became abundant. It indicates that you need to act.

- **Loss Of Energy**

Sugar is a form of energy that is easily accessible, and your body uses it as fuel. After removing all sugar from the diet, the fat becomes an energy source. Until this process happens, you will feel like you have lost your usual energy, since your body feels like something is missing.

- **Sugar Cravings**

For the first few weeks, you will always crave carb-rich foods. One of the main reasons for this is that your body is still trying to get all the energy from fat. The best solution to stop craving carbs is to increase fat intake. As your body changes, the cravings diminish accordingly, but addressing them requires mental stability.

- **Mood Swings**

One of the negative side effects of this diet is mood changes and frustration. This is mainly due to fluctuations in hormones, especially cortisol. Your body initially interprets a lack of carbs, so it will try to raise your cortisol levels and raise your blood sugar. However, this hormone is closely linked to depression and anxiety. Sudden fluctuations may make you feel sick, but they will pass in a few days.

- **Variation of the intestinal flora**

Changing the diet completely can drastically alter the intestinal microbiota (flora). In 2014, a study was conducted in which it was observed how the change of diet could alter the gut microbiota in less than 48 hours. Animal-based feeding increased the abundance of bile tolerant organisms and reduced levels of microbes that metabolize different fibers. Obviously, if the intestinal flora varies radically it can increase the chances of suffering from some type of gastrointestinal problem.

How To Deal With Possible Side Effects

1. Get Electrolyte Supplements

You can keep track of all of your nutrients, from minerals to protein and fat, but determining your electrolyte intake is a little more difficult. Salt usually has a very bad name, and most people believe that you should keep it to a minimum. It is usually good to add salt to your diet, but another option is to get an extra range of these essential minerals through supplements.

2. Get Enough Sleep

This is one thing that many people do not pay enough attention to. Adjusting your diet, especially in favor of a meat based one, can help you focus more on nutrition. However, the solution to many early symptoms is to get good sleep and even stay in the bed for an extra hour or two.

3. Never Underestimate Hydration

Trust me when I say you need to monitor your water intake in a diary.

When I first started doing this, I wondered if I was actually consuming less water. If you eat, say, three servings of food a day, I recommend that you have a pint of water during a meal and two pints in between meals.

4. BE ACTIVE AND SWEATY

Being active will obviously help you with your weight loss goals, but not just that. There are many processes in the body that are triggered by physical activity. First, exercise helps improve digestion and make it more effective. Second, it increases appetite and makes you want to eat more. More meat means more stamina, and less brain fog. Finally, the more you sweat, the better: sweat is a great way for your body to eliminate toxins that can accumulate in years of bad eating habits. Additionally, reducing toxins reduces the risk of any disease or inflammation.

5. SOLVE DIGESTIVE PROBLEMS

There is a possibility that you will experience digestive problems which, unfortunately, can be the most annoying of all. Personally, I found it harder to survive for several days with brain fog and low energy. Some of the people I spoke to suffered from flatulence and constipation for years before trying the carnivore diet.

But the most common problem here is diarrhea. This is because the gallbladder does not produce enough bile to handle the increased cholesterol. Part of it passes undigested. Yes, you guessed it, this leads to an era you don't want to be in more than a few steps from the bathroom. One option is to reduce your fat intake, which is the opposite of what I suggest in this book. Take supplements to find a better solution.

6. EAT MORE MEAT

It is not unusual to feel hungry in the first weeks, and the last thing to do is to ignore it. You can do one of two things: eat more meat or eat better quality meat. For example, buying grass-fed beef gives you the same high-quality nutrients, which in turn reduce hunger and carbs nostalgia. When dealing with lower energy levels, the best way to recharge yourself is to increase the calories and nutrients available from meat.

The Carnivore Diet On A Budget: 6 Tips To Save Money

There are no excuses to not try a carnivore diet for just 28 days. It will uncover issues you didn't even think you had. In many ways you can even save money, especially if you factor in the reduction of healthcare expenses for the rest of your life. Let's consider 6 tips that will make you save money when buying your delicious meat.

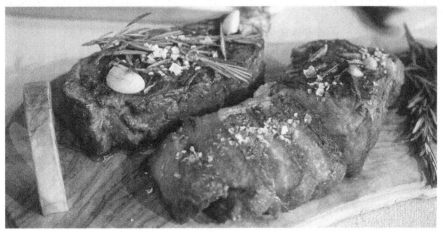

1. GO FOR GRAIN FED INSTEAD OF GRASS FED

I do think quality matters when it comes to steak. And if you can afford to pay up for great grass fed steak from a local, regenerative farm, I suggest doing so. However, it's not necessary that you get your meat from a Japanese farm where cows are hand massaged and sent to private school. The truth is that all meat is healthy — even that from cows that don't eat on an optimal diet.

The conventional carnivore diet is healthier than any other diet, regardless of the quality of your food. Most of the nutrition equation is cutting out all the crap in your existing diet. Thus, do not let perfectionism be the enemy of good. Try the carnivore diet, no matter what it takes.

Grass-fed and organic beef tend to cost much more, because they take up more space and live longer: these cows cost a lot more to their farmers. It's possible to find grass-fed beef that's fairly close to grain-fed in price — especially if you buy in bulk — but on average it will cost anywhere from 50% to 100% more.

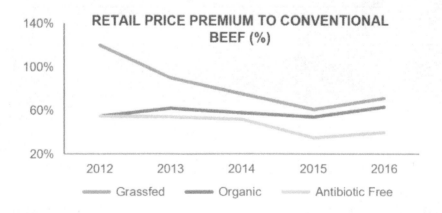

Studies show that grass-fed beef tends to contain higher levels of beta carotene, vitamin E, vitamin C and vitamin K2 than grain-fed beef. However, the levels of these vitamins in both forms of beef pale in comparison to those of other animal proteins.

Liver, for instance, has 275 times more Vitamin A than steak. Grass-fed fats like suet and tallow are superior sources of vitamin E, while liver, butter and ghee can provide more K2. Takeaway: red meat, regardless of feeding regimen, is highly nutrient-dense. Grass-fed fat is higher in nutrient concentration, but grain-fed beef tends to have more fat. Since fat stores many of these nutrients, this may even things out.

2. BUY CHEAPER CUTS OF STEAK

Within the realm of grain fed steak, you can get cheaper cuts of steak. The following cuts tend to be cheaper than your expensive ribeyes:

- **Ground beef**: You can often get this for as a cheap as $3.99 a pound.
- **Chuck roast**: Huge chunk of meat. $3 or $4. You'll want to cook this in a crock pot.
- **New York Strip**: $7 or $8 a lb.
- **Top Round**

Opting for these cuts can reduce costs significantly. Given carnivores often eat less than 1 lb of meat per sitting, you'll be getting a full meal for less than $8 on the carnivore diet. It doesn't get much cheaper than that.

3. Eat Lots Of Eggs, Beef Liver & Sardines

Three of the most nutritious foods in the worlds also happen to be the cheapest. Eggs are an absolute superfood. They're loaded with B vitamins, choline and vitamin A (retinol). And liver is like eggs on steroids.

(100g)	Blueberries	Kale	Beef	Beef Liver
Calcium	6.0 mg	72 mg	11 mg	11 mg
Phosphorus	12 mg	28 mg	140 mg	476 mg
Potassium	77 mg	228 mg	370 mg	380 mg
Iron	0.3 mg	0.9 mg	3.3 mg	8.8 mg
Zinc	0.2 mg	0.2 mg	4.4 mg	4.0 mg
Vitamin A	None	None	40 IU	53,400 IU
Vitamin D	None	None	Trace	19 IU
Vitamin E	0.6 mg	0.9 mg	1.7 mg	.63 mg
Vitamin C	9.7 mg	41 mg	None	27 mg
Niacin	0.4 mg	0.5 mg	4.0 mg	17 mg
Vitamin B6	0.1 mg	0.1 mg	.07 mg	.73 mg
Vitamin B12	None	None	1.8 mcg	111 mg
Folate	6 mcg	13 mcg	4.0 mcg	145 mcg

So 12 pasture raised eggs will run you around $6, while 1 lb of grass fed beef liver is $4 – $8. Sardines and mackerel are very cheap, too, and loaded with nutrients like selenium, bioavailable DHA, Vitamin D, iodine and Vitamin B12. Wild planet sardines cost around $3.50 for 4 oz.

4. BUY ON SALE

Grocery stores frequently run sales. And hopefully the world goes more vegan so that meat eaters will get more meat for themselves.

5. FIND A LOCAL FARM AND BUY IN BULK

One of my favorite ways to do the carnivore diet on a budget is to build a relationship with a local farm and buy in bulk from them. That way you can both support a grass-fed ranch and eat on a budget. Eat Wild has compiled over 1400 farms. It's a bit of a manual process, but you can contact farms in your area and inquire about prices. If you order with a few friends, you may be able to get an even bigger discount.

6. EAT LOTS OF SUET

Suet is extremely satiating and will cut down how much overall food you eat. I eat suet to satiation before I eat muscle meat, which helps me to burn fat and feel more satiated throughout the day. Yes, paradoxically, eating more fat can help you burn more fat. Plus you can become friends with a local butcher and often get these trimmings for free or for just $1 or $2 a pound. It's tasty and nutritious, packed with fat soluble vitamins. Tallow is another great option to add fats to your diet.

Frequently Asked Questions

WHAT CAN I EAT?

- Stage 1: only animals/meat: goat, beef, lamb, deer, small oily fish, and seafood.
- Stage 2: for people with mild or moderate digestive problems or inflammation: shellfish, beef, venison, lamb, goat, offal, fish, egg yolk.
- Stage 3: goat, duck, beef, pork, lamb, whole eggs, venison, chicken, seafood, turkey, salted meat, offal, fish
- Fatty dairy products - if acceptable.

HOW MUCH MEAT SHOULD I EAT PER DAY?

The Carnivore diet is not a calorie counting diet. It is an elimination diet designed to remove inflammatory foods and other ingredients that modern nutrition has introduced. You should eat until you're full or until your calorie goal (if you have one) is reached. It's ultimately up to you. The only tip that was helpful for me is to eat sufficient fat. If you find yourself with an insatiable hunger, you may not be eating enough fat. If this is you, try eating fat first to satiation, then adding in the muscle meat after. Most people end up eating 1-2 lbs of meat a day.

HOW MANY TIMES SHOULD I EAT?

The beauty of the carnivore diet lies in its simplicity. Eat when you are hungry and do not eat when you are not hungry. This allows you to reconnect with your body — no need to count calories or macros. You will not be hungry. If you use fat instead of carbohydrates, you do not need to eat often. In addition, when you are hungry, you are not craving, you do not have blood sugar or the energy oppressed by carbohydrates. Do not worry if you are a little hungry and do not find what suits you. You can wait to eat later. Many carnivores settle with one or two meals per day, sometimes three. You need to eat your largest and last meal of the day at least 2 hours before going to bed, or from 4 to 6 hours if you are diagnosed with a disease, preferably in the afternoon.

WHAT SNACKS CAN I EAT?

For those who like to eat small snacks during the day, it is recommended to eat sausages, small pieces of meat and small fish. However, if your goal is weight loss I recommend that you avoid unnecessary snacking. If you eat enough appropriate food during your main meals, you don't need to snack.

CAN I EAT PROCESSED MEATS?

No. Grass-fed animal products should be the only food source you consume. Processed meats like pepperoni and other lunch meats typically contain harmful ingredients, like artificial nitrates to preserve its shelf life, which can negatively impact your health.

DOES THE CARNIVORE DIET PUT YOU IN KETOSIS?

While ketosis isn't the direct goal, it often occurs while following the carnivore diet. This is because the diet aims for zero-carbs, so by design your body will begin to prioritize burning fat over carbs and sugars.

HOW LONG IS THE ADAPTATION PERIOD?

Around 1 month. If you're like most people, you've been eating carbohydrates your whole life, so your body will take some time to adjust.

DO I GET ALL THE NUTRIENTS I NEED?

In short, yes. While some oppose it, it has become clear that the recommended daily allowances of various vitamins and minerals are all based on carbohydrate consumption and that meat-based foods have changed these rules. First of all, adopting a meat-based diet increases intestinal absorption, so the nutrients you take in have greater power in the body, while carbohydrates compete with different nutrients, reducing their effectiveness. This is particularly the case with vitamin C. It is said that a certain amount of vitamin C is needed to prevent scurvy (10 mg per day), but scurvy has not been found in carnivores that have been following the diet for decades. Do not take vitamin C or any other supplements. Meat, especially organs, contains a small amount of vitamin C, but without carbohydrates in the diet it is enough. Longtime hunters who eat good fresh meat don't seem to have any malnutrition.

DO I REALLY NEED FIBER?

This is one of my favorite topics. This is because people who eat other foods, especially vegetarians, often want to use this as a first attack. Fiber is mainly indigestible cellulose, which cleans the intestines, destroys the mucous membranes, and prevents the absorption of nutrients from the rest of the food. If you don't eat a lot of junk food, you don't need too much fiber.

IS RED MEAT BAD FOR ME?

As with many things about nutrition and life, you need to

consider other variables before drawing a conclusion. As long as you don't exercise and eat lots of sugar and lean meat, you will not be very healthy. However, eating lean meats, exercising, avoiding sugar, and eating other healthy foods can be great.

WHAT ABOUT FAT?

There is a controversy that meat fat causes too much body fat. There are so many variables that affect fat, and they all concern our body. If you are eating a lot of fat and sugar, this is very different from eating a lot of fat without sugar. Sugar causes problems, not fat. Exercise is also an important factor.

WILL IT WORK FOR ATHLETES?

Yes. Many fitness enthusiasts assume that glucose from carbs is the best source for quick and immediate energy to fuel workouts and competition. On the carnivore diet, your body will go through a process called gluconeogenesis where some protein is converted into just enough glucose for certain body functions.

Can You Build Muscle On The Carnivore Diet?

While it has to be supplemented with working out, of course! Many people quote muscle growth as a result of going carnivore. This is due to an increase in average protein intake.

4-Week Carnivore Diet Meal Plan

The goal with this plan will be to transition you from more variety in meat to less, while still cutting out the inflammatory foods. When you start the carnivore diet it's very common to experience gut issues like diarrhea and constipation. But think of this like burning off the deadwood. Growth always comes with pain. Don't let these pains stop you.

With that being said, this meal plan is formulated to minimize the gut pain you experience. My philosophy is to just jump right in and go cold turkey on the vegetables and carbohydrates. If you're addicted to something, it doesn't make sense to have a little bit of it. You don't tell an alcoholic it's okay to have a shot of vodka before bed.

However, when it comes to meat, you may want to try starting with more variety so that you don't quit out of boredom as you transition. Over time, however, you'll come to love beef and most cravings can and should go away.

WEEK 1: DIET PLAN AND SHOPPING LIST

I advise people starting on the carnivore diet to take a 3-level approach elimination way of eating. Basically, over several weeks, you work towards a beef only diet. You see how this is different from many common plant-based or low-carb diet.

For the 4-week carnivore diet meal plan, I will gradually change the meat selection to get you to level 3 by the end of the week. The first mistake to avoid, and something you will notice below, is that you shouldn't stay away from fats or fatty meat.

Saturated fat is not your enemy, and there are increasing studies that show that sugar is to blame when it comes to heart disease.

You will notice that in the first week of this carnivore diet meal plan I included some dairy products for you to eat. This will help you adjust and stay focused during the initial stages of your diet, until you complete the transition.

Remember that you must have one pint of drinking water with every meal as well as at least one pint of water in between meals. One pint is equivalent to 470 mL, leading to a total of at least five pints (2400 mL) of water per day.

When I shop, I open up an excel and map out how many meals I plan to eat of a certain food and the amount per meal, so I am able to calculate the total amount to bulk buy.

WEEK 1	Breakfast	Lunch	Dinner
Monday	• Five slices of bacon (about 4 ounces) • one or two 100% pork sausages (3 ounces)	• Grilled beef burger patty only (10 ounces) with a slice of cheese	• Four fresh racks of lamb (12 ounces)
Tuesday	• 3 grilled 100% pork sausages (5 ounces) • 3 slices of bacon (4 ounces)	• Roasted salmon cutlets on the bone (15 ounces) with butter	• Grilled porterhouse steak (12 ounces) with butter
Wednesday	• Grilled trout fillets (10 ounces) with butter	• Roasted pork belly (10 ounces)	• Slow roast topside of beef (12 ounces)
Thursday	• Grilled ground beef burger patty (8 ounces) with cheese	• Roast salmon cutlets on the bone (15 ounces) with butter	• Grilled porterhouse steak (12 ounces)
Friday	• 2 grilled chicken breasts with skin (8 ounces)	• Grilled trout fillets (16 ounces)	• Slow roast topside of beef (12 ounces)
Saturday	• 3 grilled 100% pork sausages (5 ounces) • 3 slices of bacon (4 ounces)	• 4 fresh lamb chops (12 ounces)	• Grilled ribeye steak (12 ounces)
Sunday	• 2 grilled chicken breasts with skin (8 ounces)	• 4 pork chops fried or grilled (12 ounces)	• Grilled ribeye steak (12 ounces)

Shopping list for the week:

- Bacon: 12 ounces
- 100% pork sausages: 13 ounces
- Pork chops: 12 ounces
- Pork belly: 10 ounces
- Lamb Chops: 24 ounces
- Chicken breasts: 16 ounces
- Beef (Grounded): 18 ounces
- Porterhouse steak: 24 ounces
- Ribeye steak: 24 ounces
- Topside of beef 24 ounces
- Salmon cutlets: 30 ounces (or other fatty fish)
- Trout: 26 ounces
- Butter: 1 lbs
- Cheese: 1/2 lbs

WEEK 2: DIET PLAN AND SHOPPING LIST

During the second week of our carnivore diet, we're going to be removing most of the milk byproducts. We'll still allow some butter to be used in cooking, but dairy foods like cheese should be gone by now.

I would also suggest that you start experimenting a little with the way you're eating meat. For the beef, move to the rare side of cooking as this will preserve high amounts of nutritional values.

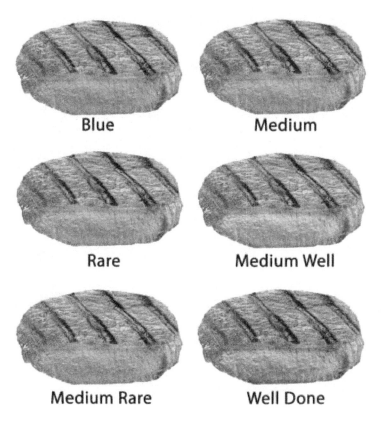

Blue   Medium

Rare   Medium Well

Medium Rare   Well Done

The more you cook these, the more of the protein, nutrient, minerals, and vitamins break down. We'll still be keeping a mix of seafood, poultry, pork, lamb, and grass-fed beef, but we'll add in some organ meat as well.

WEEK 2	Breakfast	Lunch	Dinner
Monday	• 2 grilled chicken breasts with skin (8 ounces)	• Slow roast topside of beef (12 ounces)	• 4 fresh lamb chops (12 ounces)
Tuesday	• Grilled ground beef burger patty (8 ounces)	• Roast salmon cutlets on the bone (15 ounces)	• Grilled ribeye steak (8 ounces) • Roasted beef liver (4 ounces)
Wednesday	• 5 slices of bacon (about 4 ounces) • 1 or two 100% pork sausages (3 ounces)	• Grilled porterhouse steak (12 ounces) with butter	• Slow roast topside of beef (12 ounces)
Thursday	• Grilled ribeye steak (12 ounces)	• 3 grilled chicken breasts with skin (12 ounces)	• Grilled ground beef burger patty (12 ounces)
Friday	• Grilled sirloin steak (8 ounces) with butter	• Slow roast topside of beef (8 ounces) • Roasted beef liver (4 ounces)	• 4 pork chops fried or grilled (12 ounces)
Saturday	• Grilled ground beef burger patty (8 ounces)	• Roast salmon cutlets on the bone (15 ounces) with butter	• Grilled sirloin steak (12 ounces)
Sunday	• Grilled ribeye steak (8 ounces)	• Slow roast topside of beef (12 ounces)	• 3 grilled chicken breasts with skin (12 ounces) • Roasted beef liver (4 ounces)

Some people starting on a carnivore diet may be a bit squeamish about this, but if you look up the nutrients they contain, you might change your mind. These are a few things to consider if you don't want to try organ meats.

You may also ask your butcher to cut them into slices. I personally found this helped initially, as it will just look like any other cut of meat.

Shopping list for the week:

- Chicken breasts: 32 ounces
- Topside of beef: 44 ounces
- Lamb chops: 12 ounces
- Salmon cutlets : 30 ounces (or other fatty fish)
- Ribeye steak: 28 ounces
- Ribeye steak: 24 ounces
- 100% pork sausages: 3 ounces
- Porterhouse steak: 12 ounces
- Pork chops: 12 ounces
- Beef's liver: 12 ounces

WEEK 3: DIET PLAN AND SHOPPING LIST

For the third week of the carnivore diet, we're removing all the milk byproducts left, and we'll slightly increase the shift towards cow's meat. You'll notice that there are fewer meals covered by fish and poultry, and we'll even add in a beef-only day in preparation for next week.

At this stage, you should also be eating your grass-fed beef at least medium-rare to get most of the vitamin, protein, and micronutrient benefits. You will have cooked many kinds of beef and should be getting used to judging it better.

What you can also do is cut your steaks in half and then cook one part medium-rare and the other medium-well. One thing you should notice is that there is a lot more flavor to the medium-rare part, even with just salt to season. You can opt to use a smoker box as well for added flavor.

We're also introducing a bit more organ meat into the mix. Eating organ parts is highly beneficial to balance your efforts when on an animal meat carnivore diet, even though they are lower in fat. From one serving of eating liver or kidney, you can get more nutrient and vitamins, especially Vitamin B12 and Vitamin A, than most plant foods, and it's more than your daily needs. Also, the raw liver does contain some Vitamin C. You won't believe the nutrition these organs can give to the body.

WEEK 3	Breakfast	Lunch	Dinner
Monday	• Grilled Beef (Grounded) burger patty (8 ounces)	• Slow roast topside of beef (8 ounces) • Roasted beef liver (4 ounces)	• Roast salmon (or other fatty fish) cutlets on the bone (15 ounces)
Tuesday	• 5 slices of bacon (about 4 ounces) • One or two 100% pork sausages (3 ounces)	• Grilled ground beef burger patty (12 ounces)	• Grilled porterhouse steak (12 ounces)
Wednesday	• Grilled ribeye steak (8 ounces)	• Grilled ground beef burger patty (12 ounces)	• 4 pork chops fried or grilled (12 ounces)
Thursday	• Grilled porterhouse steak (8 ounces)	• 3 grilled chicken breasts with skin (12 ounces)	• Slow roast topside of beef (8 ounces) • Slow cooked beef Kidney (4 ounces)
Friday	• Grilled ground beef burger patty (8 ounces)	• Grilled ribeye steak (8 ounces) • Roasted beef liver (4 ounces)	• Grilled porterhouse steak (12 ounces)
Saturday	• 3 fresh lamb chops (8 ounces)	• Grilled ground beef burger patty (12 ounces)	• Slow roast topside of beef (12 ounces)
Sunday	• Grilled ribeye steak (8 ounces)	• Grilled ground beef burger patty (12 ounces)	• Slow roast topside of beef (8 ounces) • Slow cooked beef Kidney (4 ounces)

87

Shopping list for the week:

- Chicken breasts: 12 ounces
- Topside of beef: 36 ounces
- Lamb chops: 8 ounces
- Salmon cutlets: 15 ounces
- Ribeye steak: 24 ounces
- Bacon: 4 ounces
- 100% pork sausages: 3 ounces
- Porterhouse steak: 32 ounces
- Beef's liver: 8 ounces
- Beef Kidney: 8 ounces

WEEK 4: DIET PLAN AND SHOPPING LIST

If you've made it this far on the carnivore diet, then you can start looking forward to noticing some health benefits. You should be feeling a lot more active physically with increased levels of concentrations as a result of your metabolism having entirely shifted to ketosis and blood sugar levels remaining stable. This is what happens to your body when you undergo the ketogenic diet.

Some people even experience blood sugar drop while on the carnivore diet because the carbohydrate intake is not right. This must be a precaution to people with Type 2 Diabetes. You should also find those high carbohydrates cravings will have reduced because you're now better equipped to get all the energy you need from fat and protein.

This week, we'll be removing all meat that doesn't come from cows. You'll also notice that we're adding organ meat on a more regular basis in the all-meat diet. And there is one other thing that you should try and factor in for this week.

All the meat you buy should come from grass-fed only cows, and this will also add more healthy fats. It doesn't have to be organic fat, but that is an option if you can afford it. If your budget doesn't stretch to this, try to add in as much grass-fed cow's meat when you can.

Also, because there are limited recipes to follow on a high-protein and high-fat carnivore diet, you should try and vary your cooking techniques. I find grilling your meat is a great way to get some of the charred flavors of animal fat.

WEEK 4	Breakfast	Lunch	Dinner
Monday	• Grilled Beef (Grounded) burger patty (8 ounces)	• Slow roast topside of beef (8 ounces) • Roasted beef liver (4 ounces) one pinch of salt	• BBQ beef ribs (24 ounces including bones)
Tuesday	• Grilled sirloin steak (8 ounces)	• BBQ ground beef burger patty (12 ounces)	• Grilled porterhouse steak (12 ounces)
Wednesday	• Grilled ribeye steak (8 ounces)	• Grilled ground beef burger patty (8 ounces) • Roasted beef liver (4 ounces)	• BBQ sirloin steak (12 ounces)
Thursday	• Grilled porterhouse steak (8 ounces)	• BBQ beef ribs (24 ounces including bones)	• Slow roast topside of beef (8 ounces) • Slow cooked beef Kidney (4 ounces)
Friday	• Grilled ground beef burger patty (8 ounces)	• BBQ ribeye steak (12 ounces)	• Grilled porterhouse steak (12 ounces)
Saturday	• Grilled ground beef burger patty (8 ounces) • Slow cooked beef Kidney (4 ounces)	• Slow roast topside of beef (12 ounces)	• BBQ beef ribs (24 ounces including bones)
Sunday	• Grilled ribeye steak (8 ounces)	• BBQ ground beef burger patty (12 ounces)	• Slow roast topside of beef (8 ounces) • Slow cooked beef Kidney (4 ounces)

Shopping list for the week:

- Topside of beef: 36 ounces
- Beef (Grounded): 56 ounces
- Ribeye steak: 28 ounces
- Porterhouse steak: 32 ounces
- Beef liver: 8 ounces

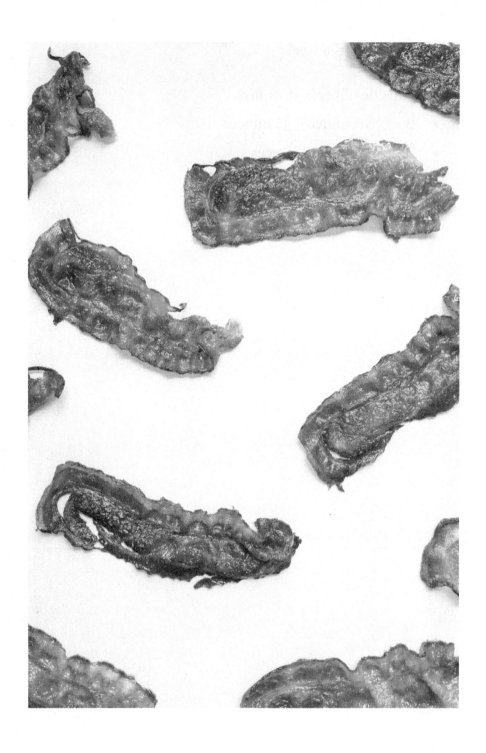

Recipes

With these carnivore diet recipes, there's no longer any excuse not to try the carnivore diet. One of the most common concerns is that there's not enough variety. People think they'll get tired of just eating seared steak every night. But these options eliminate those concerns. Here are my 10 favorite carnivore diet recipes when I'm looking to change things up.

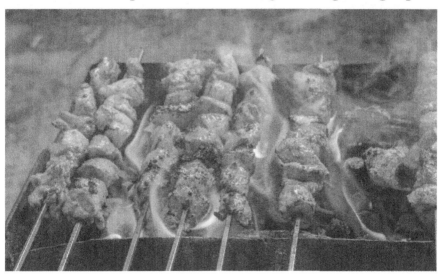

1. CARNIVORE WAFFLES

You can make waffles entirely from animal products. They are extremely tasty and easy to make. Here's how.

Ingredients

- Ground beef
- Salt
- A fat: ghee, butter or tallow
- Eggs
- Blender and waffle maker

Recipe

1. Add meat, eggs and salt to a blender. Blend it up until smooth. I recommend 8oz ground beef and 6 eggs.
2. Spread batter on a waffle maker.
3. Cook until complete.

2. STEAK TARTARE

Here's how I make it. Use a leaner cut of steak for this.

1. Cut steak into 1-inch cubes and put in the freezer for 10 minutes.
2. Break 2-3 eggs (I just use egg yolks). Mix with the steak in a bowl.
3. Chop steak as fine as you'd like.
4. Form it together like a steak hockey puck.

3. Crock Pot Stew (Carnivore Salad)

This is what I call carnivore salad. One of my favorite things to do on the carnivore diet when I'm lazy is to chuck all sorts of different meats into a crock pot or slow cooker: Steak, shrimp, pork, bacon...Try it out!

4. Beef Liver Pate

Beef liver is packed with the most important nutrients for your brain, immune system and metabolism. But the problem is to make it appetizing. This beef liver pate recipe is one of my favorite ways to add it to my diet.

Ingredients

- Beef liver
- Sea salt
- Ghee, butter or cream

Recipe

1. Cut beef liver into 1 inch strips.
2. Saute in a pan on medium-high heat until it's almost cooked all the way through.
3. Transfer liver to a food processor.
4. Blend with cream, ghee or butter until it's a smooth consistency.

5. Refrigerate and chill in mason jars.

5. BONE BROTH

Bone broth is one of the most nutritious foods in the world. Bone marrow and cartilage is loaded with fat soluble nutrients like Vitamin A and DHA. Connective tissue is also very high in glycine, which is important for collagen synthesis and methylation. Some studies have shown that glutamine, an amino acid in the gelatin, can help to heal your gut. This isn't a meal per se, but it's a great addition to the carnivore diet.

Ingredients

- 1 gallon of water
- 2 tbsp (30 ml) apple cider vinegar
- 4 lbs of marrow bones
- Salt

Recipe

1. Place all ingredients in a large pot or slow cooker.
2. If in a pot, bring to a simmer.
3. Cook for 12–24 hours. The longer it cooks, the better.
4. Strain into a container.

6. Pork Rinds

Pork cracklings are one of my favorite high fat snacks on the carnivore diet. They're also a great way to get some crunch back into your life, which I know many of you carnivores are missing. You're going to need to find a local butcher that can sell pork skin for this (if you're a carnivore this shouldn't be a problem as I'm sure you have a butcher that's your best friend already).

1. Trim the fat off the skin.
2. Cut the skin into 1 inch blocks.
3. Place them on a parchment lined baking sheet skin side up.
4. Sprinkle each piece with salt to taste.
5. Bake at 325 °F until crispy. This usually takes 1-2 hours.

7. Carnivore Sausage

This is another recipe that requires some equipment, but is well worth the effort. All it takes is a meat grinder, which you can get for $30 or so and is definitely worth it. I used to love sausage, but unfortunately most of them have fillings and other toxins. I like to combine ground beef, with bacon and egg yolks to make mine.

Here's my recipe:

1. Use 2:1 beef to bacon ratio.
2. Cut bacon into 1 inch slices.
3. Put into meat grinder. Combine with ground beef in a bowl.
4. Add 4 egg yolks for every 1lb of meat. Mix in bowl with sea salt.
5. Put back into the meat grinder and connect the casing to the end of it and crank it in.
6. Let the sausage come out in one long coil. Make sure to leave 6-10 inches at the end. Twist the completed sausage stick every 6 inches or so into individual sausages.
7. Cook at 400 degrees for 30 minutes.

8. ORGAN BURGERS

Here's another of my favorite ways to sneak more organs into your life. I usually do this with a combo of heart, liver and ground beef in a 25/25/50 ratio.

1. Grind the liver & heart into ¼ inch pieces.
2. Combine with ground beef.
3. Melt butter or ghee.
4. Mix everything together with the butter in a bowl. Add in sea salt.
5. Shape into burgers.

6. Bake for 25 minutes at 250 degrees.

7. Optional: Add minced bacon.

9. BRISKET

Brisket is the king of braised beef. It takes the most care to cook, but like a fine wine comes out much better with time. It's simple, but one of my favorites to change it up from cuts of steak. Brisket is tough, but once you get through its outer shell it turns into the richest, most tender meat you can eat. My favorite way to cook it is in a slow cooker for 12 hours in some bone broth.

10. DEHYDRATED BEEF LIVER JERKY

Liver jerky is an energy packed snack, high in protein and actually makes liver taste good.

1. Slice beef liver as thin as desired.

2. Sea salt both sides.

3. Dehydrate in a dehydrator to desired crispiness.

Did you like this book?

If yes, please spread the love and leave a positive review on Amazon, to help other people discover it.

Thanks!

Paul Baker

Made in United States
Orlando, FL
19 March 2025

59633616R10056